looking back at ...

The Beatles

Published by Cognitive Books Limited,
115 New Road, Croxley Green WD3 3EN. United Kingdom
Published by Cognitive Books, 2024

Text © Matt Singleton, 2024
Illustrations © Simon Reid, 2024,
except illustration on page 62 © Samuel Larn, 2024

ISBN: 978-1-7384591-0-0

This book has primarily been developed and published for those living with dementia and their loved ones. This is not intended to be an official history of The Beatles. However, every attempt has been made to research the topic thoroughly and any inaccuracies are unintentional.

We are committed to working with print partners who prioritise environmental and social responsibility. Printed and bound in Latvia by PNB Print.

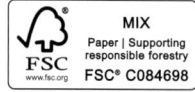

www.cognitivebooks.co.uk

looking back at ...
The Beatles

Written by Matt Singleton

Illustrations by Simon Reid

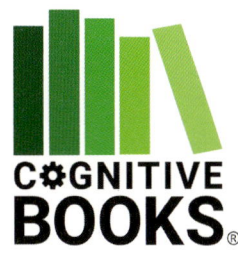

COGNITIVE
BOOKS®

 Download the free audio version of this book – read by world-famous actor, Bill Nighy – at cognitivebooks.co.uk/download or by scanning the QR code.

If you're the supporter (e.g. a carer or a loved one) of the person reading this book, you can enjoy it too! There are some useful hints and tips for you at the back of this Cognitive Book to make sure everyone gets the most out of it.

Become a Cognitive Bookworm at cognitivebooks.co.uk

This book has been created in collaboration with Alzheimer's Society. 5% of the publisher's proceeds from the sale of this Cognitive Book will be paid to the charity. The aim of Cognitive Books is to increase this contribution over time.

You can find lots of useful information to support people living with dementia at alzheimers.org.uk

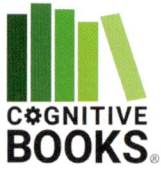

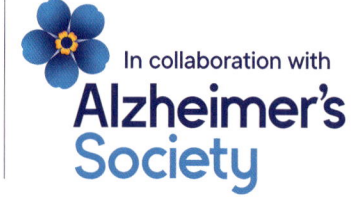

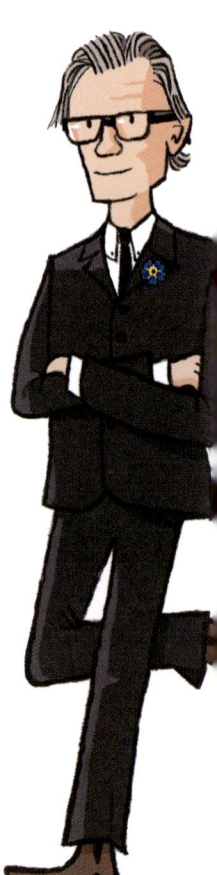

For my Dad, Brian, and his wife, Colleen:
With love from me to you.

With special thanks to Ella, Lindsey, Graeme, Michelle, Tash and the team at Alzheimer's Society, Simon, Bill, Daisy, Ross, Sam, Robyn, Sarah, Neil, the PCG team, Nicky, Nicola, Jai, Gill, Adelina, Ros, my colleagues at Swiss Re and – as always – Claire, William, Ben and (of course) Smidge The Cat.

Matt Singleton, 2023

—

In loving memory
Matthew Chapman
1974-2023

Contents

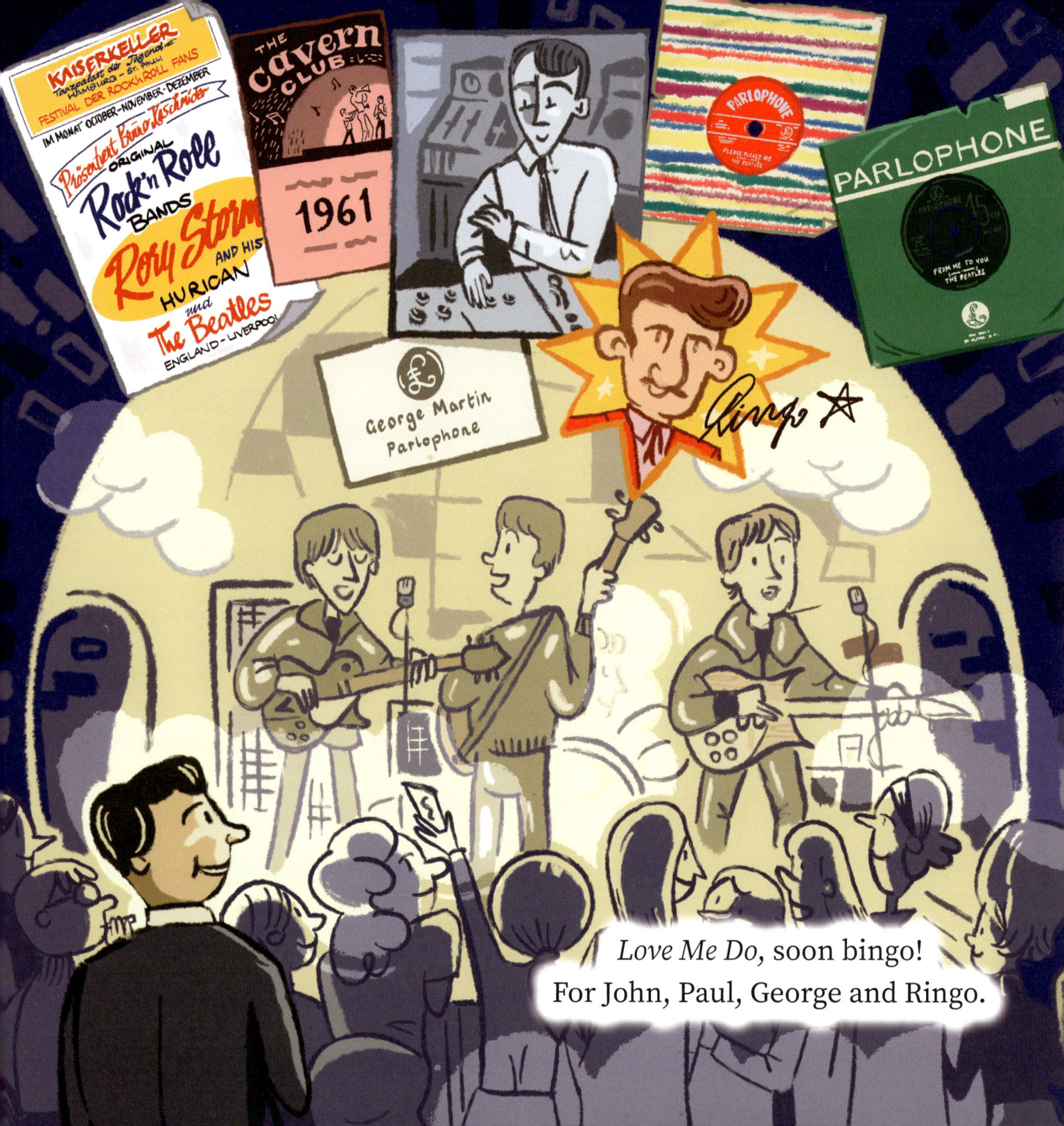

Love Me Do, soon bingo!
For John, Paul, George and Ringo.

1960 to 1963

Back to sixties Hamburg, no place for a Scouse fella,
Our young lads from Liverpool play the Kaiserkeller.
What they'd become they couldn't know, we never quite recovered,
Epstein's watching at The Cavern, The Beatles get discovered.
Decca make a big mistake; they see guitars departin',
At Parlophone a deal is done, produced by that George Martin!
Love Me Do, *Please Please Me*, *From Me To You* then bingo!
Everyone now knows the names of John, Paul, George and Ringo.

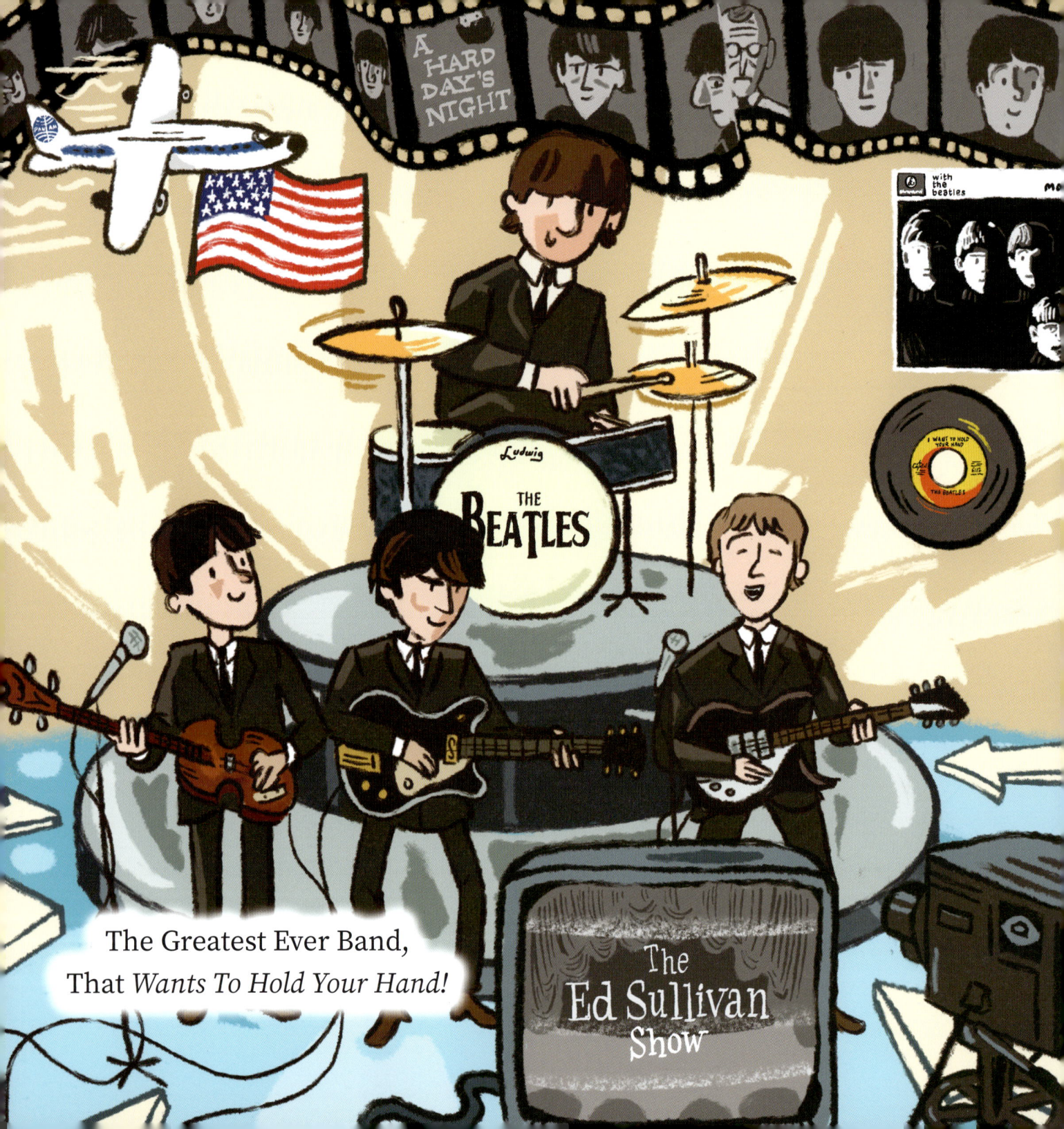

1963 to 1964

Here they come, they *Feel Fine*, adorned with mop-topped hair,
On radio, on stage, TV, it's Beatles everywhere.
America, Ed Sullivan, success is quick as lightning,
The Quarrymen are long behind now John and Paul are writing.
She Loves You makes the young girls scream, they're all so cool and groovy,
Then on they go to *A Hard Day's Night*, they've only made a movie!
Now listen *With The Beatles*, the Greatest Ever Band,
They mess about, they *Twist And Shout*, they *Want To Hold Your Hand.*

These memories last forever,
A fine old *Mystery Tour*,
Tomorrow Never Knows, my friend,
Remember our Fab Four.

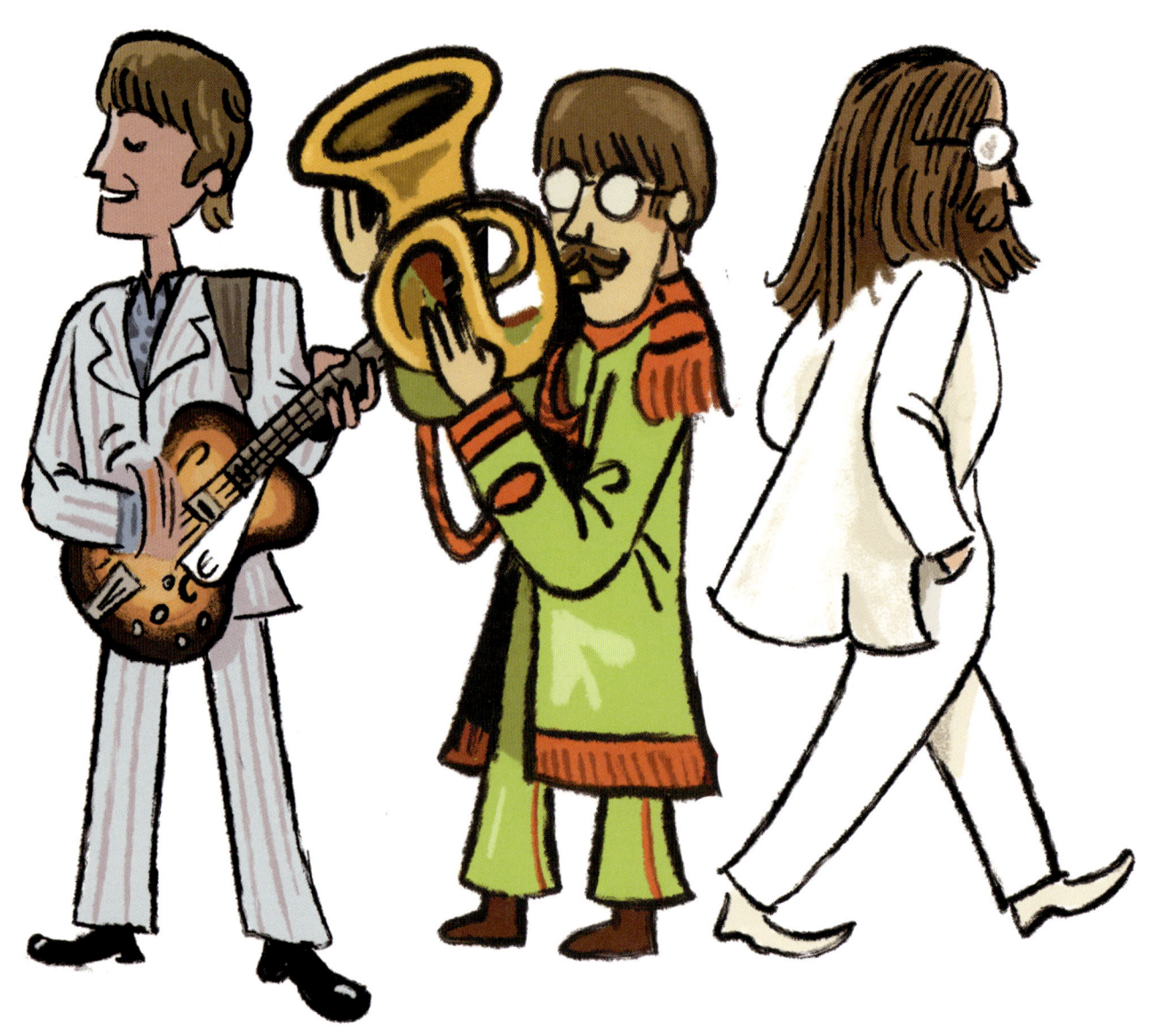

The all-round superstar,
A mean rhythm guitar!

John

That haunting voice, so profound, an all-round superstar,
A *Hero, Working Class* you know, and mean rhythm guitar.
The group's clown, John's jokey japes, the brassy brash astounder,
A son at home, those Gandhi specs, The Beatles first-come founder.
The humour and the cheekiness, they hide a darker truth,
His dad who left, mam's awful death, a tragic, painful youth.
Worse tragedy not far away; *Give Peace A Chance* we thought,
Imagine now what could have been, were his life not cut too short.

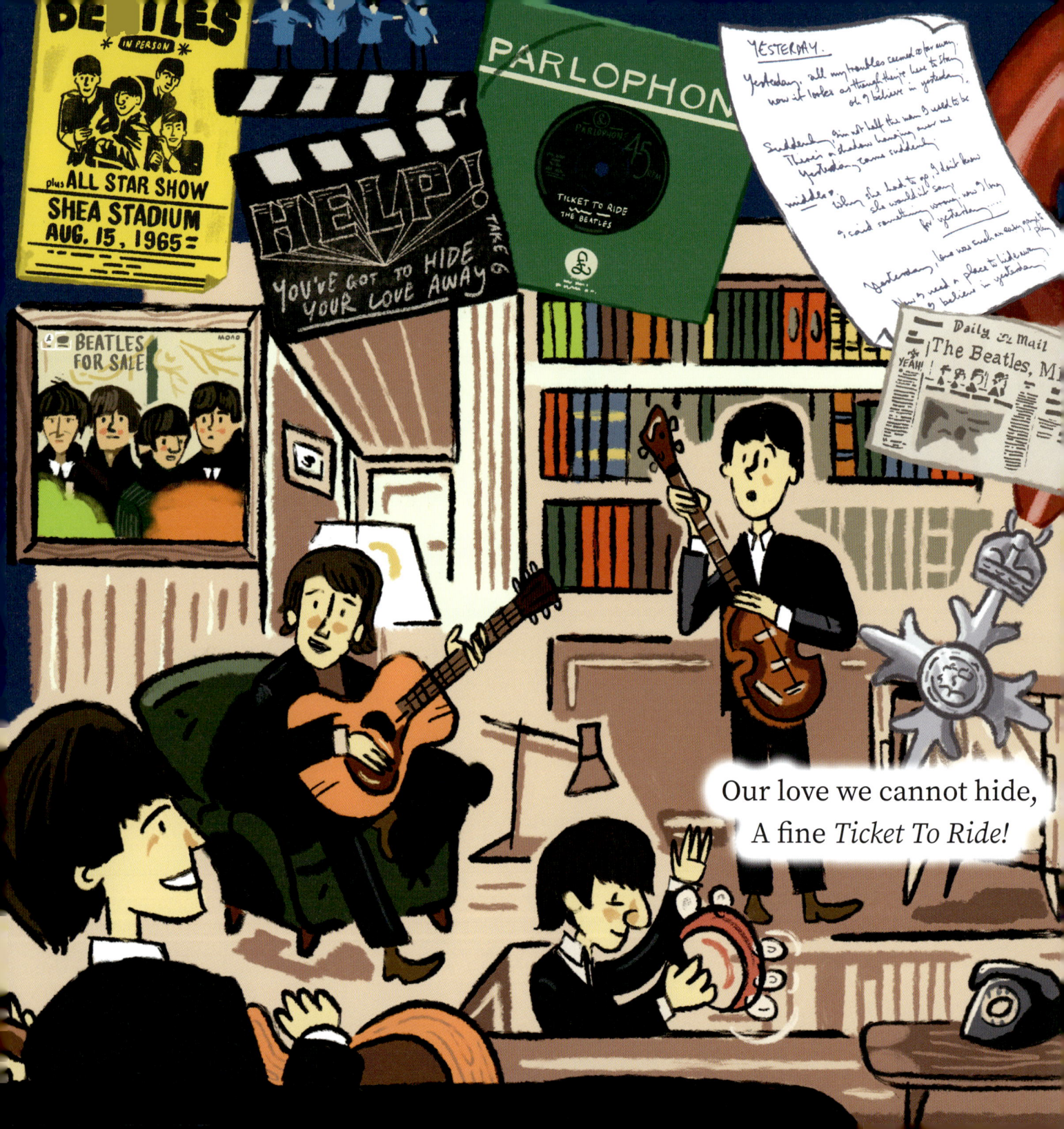

Our love we cannot hide,
A fine *Ticket To Ride!*

1964 to 1965

We Can Work It Out now, the music's oh so sleek!
A tour that never ends, working through *Eight Days A Week.*
It seems like only *Yesterday* our love we could not hide,
Help! Another film on board; a fine *Ticket To Ride.*
The *Beatles* were *For Sale*, now a money man's machine,
All four receive an MBE, they're honoured by their Queen.
The old guard and establishment question if they earned this,
But over time it mattered not, cos John went and returned his!

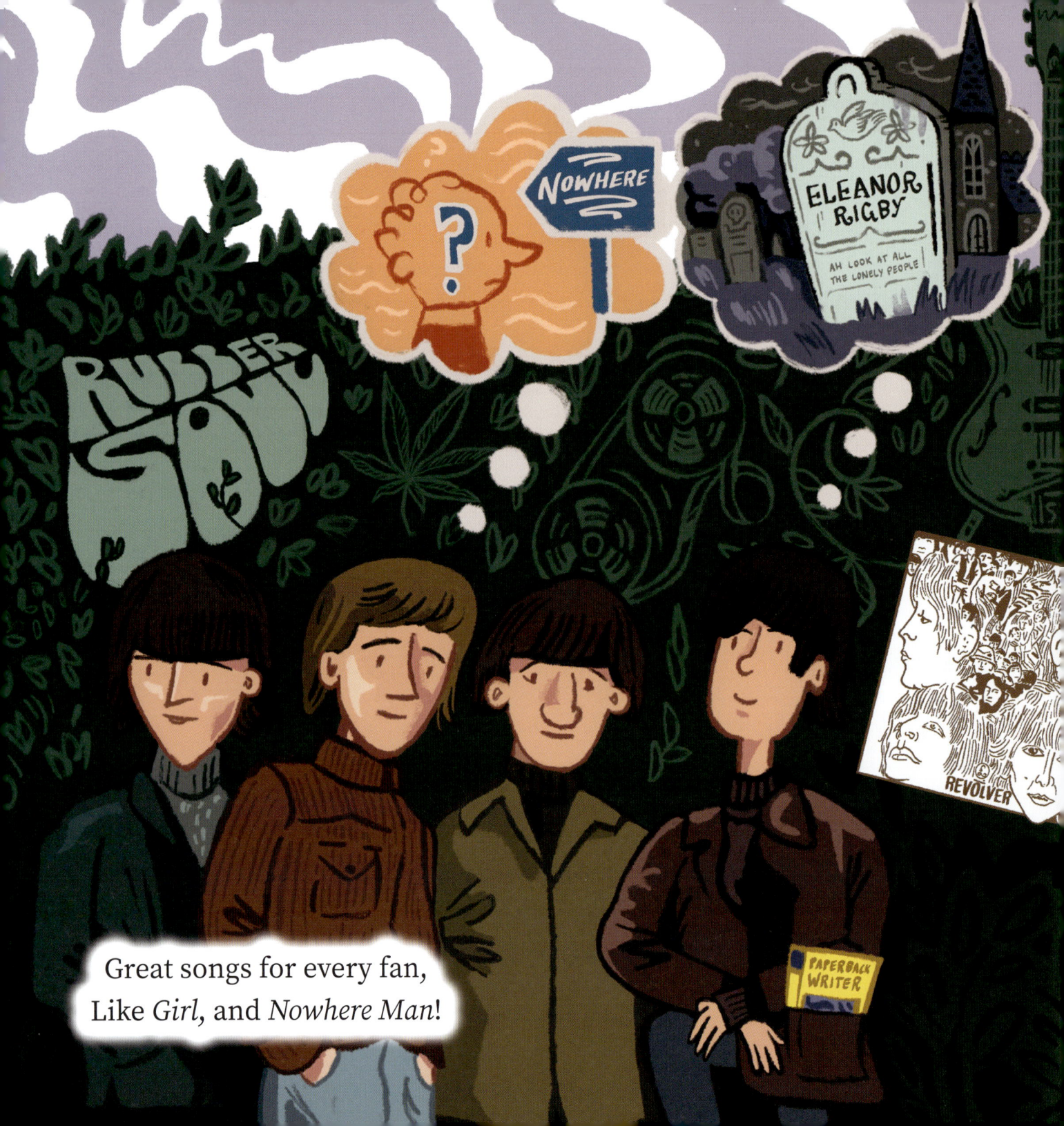

1965 to 1966

Now up a notch, another peak, the writing's beyond thrillin',
Rubber Soul, a masterpiece, with echoes of Bob Dylan.
In My Life you can *Drive My Car*, *The Word* for every fan,
Now *Girl*, *Michelle*, please listen to a real *Nowhere Man*.
Revolver takes it further now, songsmiths flaunting flair,
Paperback Writer, *Rigby* too, *Here, There, Everywhere*.
The quality is peaking, there's no sign of it abating,
These serious musicians now find playing live frustrating.

These memories last forever,
A fine old *Mystery Tour*,
For us, *Oh Darling*! *For You Blue*,
Remember our Fab Four.

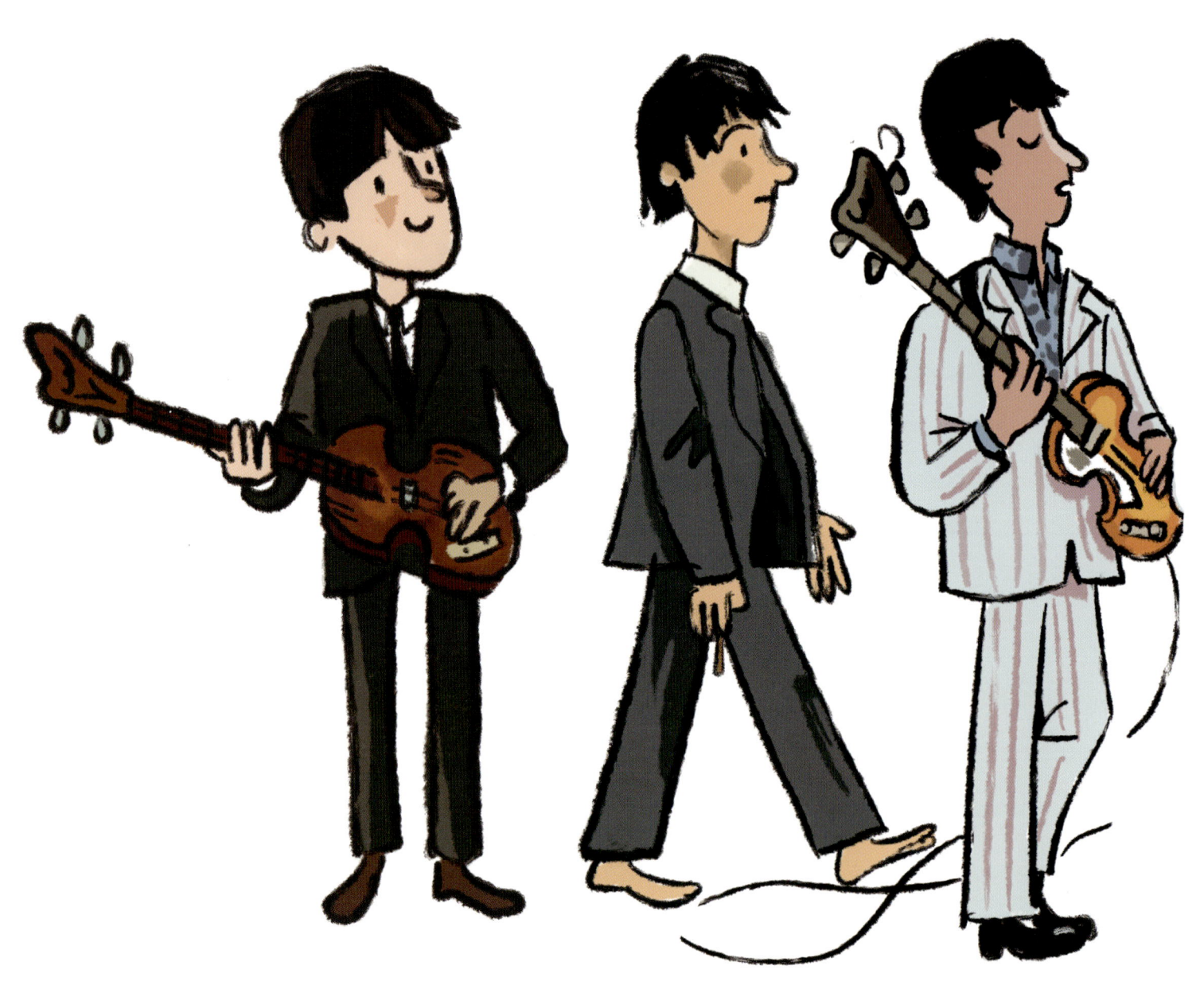

The one with a baby face,
Who plays a left-hand bass!

Paul

The melodic one, he's Mary's son, blessed with a baby face,
His talent shines, dressed to the nines, he plays a left-hand bass.
A versatile musician: piano, drums or lead,
Though did you know he plays by ear? Sheet music he can't read.
An amazing future beckons, with booming voice he sings,
Best forget *The Froggy Song* and focus on the Wings!
But if you were to meet him, on terms that are first names,
It's your call, the mid-name's Paul, McCartney's really James.

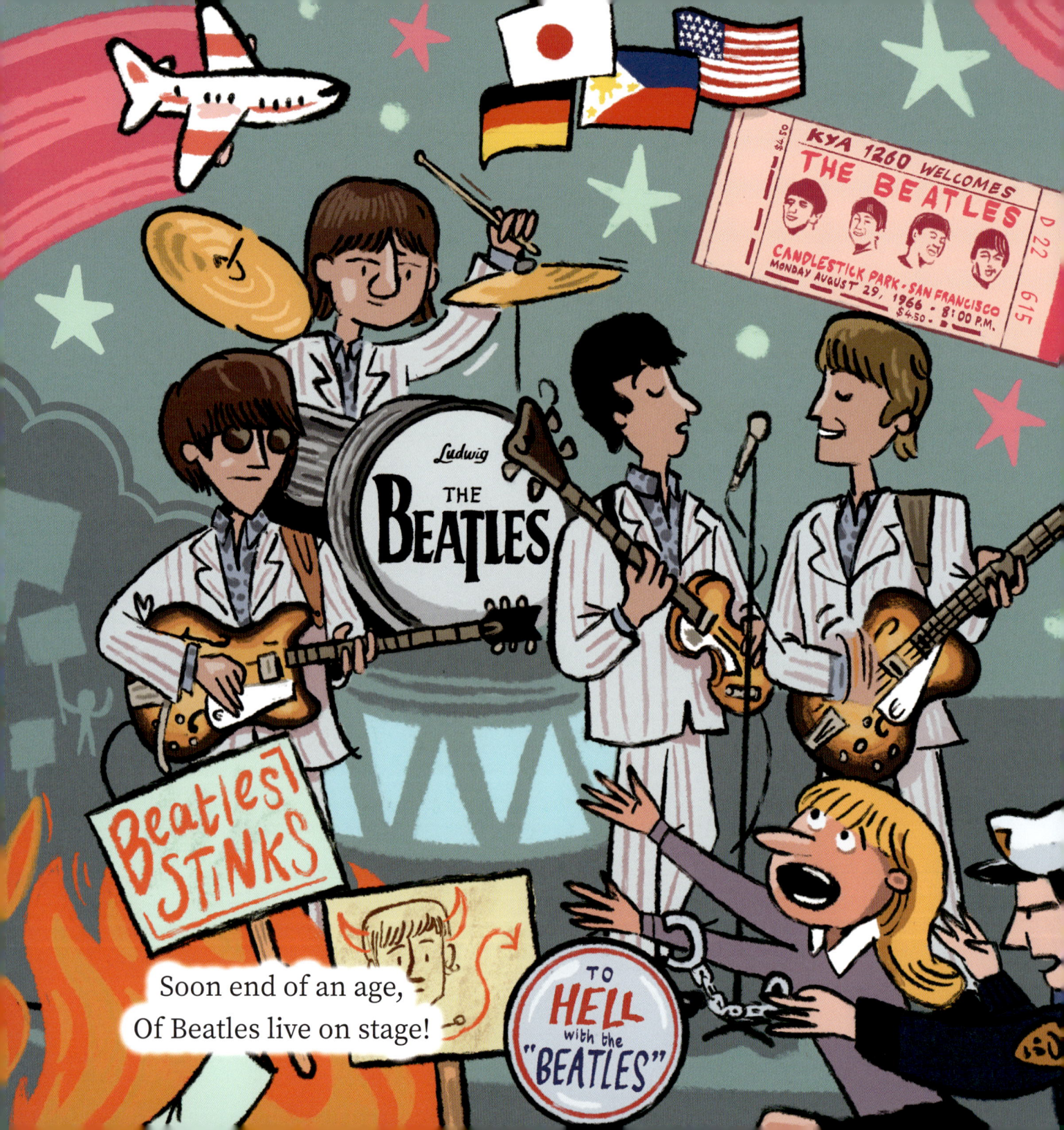

Soon end of an age,
Of Beatles live on stage!

The end of touring

The spotlight and the screaming begin to take their toll,
Controversy follows with their *Music (Rock And Roll)*.
Philippines, Shea Stadium, soon end of the age,
An era when we could see The Beatles live on stage.
A final tour, in USA, a newspaper press hire,
Heard John compare hysteria to that of The Messiah.
'Bigger than Christ' (the headline ran), records burnt in dark,
And soon enough the lights go down on Candlestick's Ballpark.

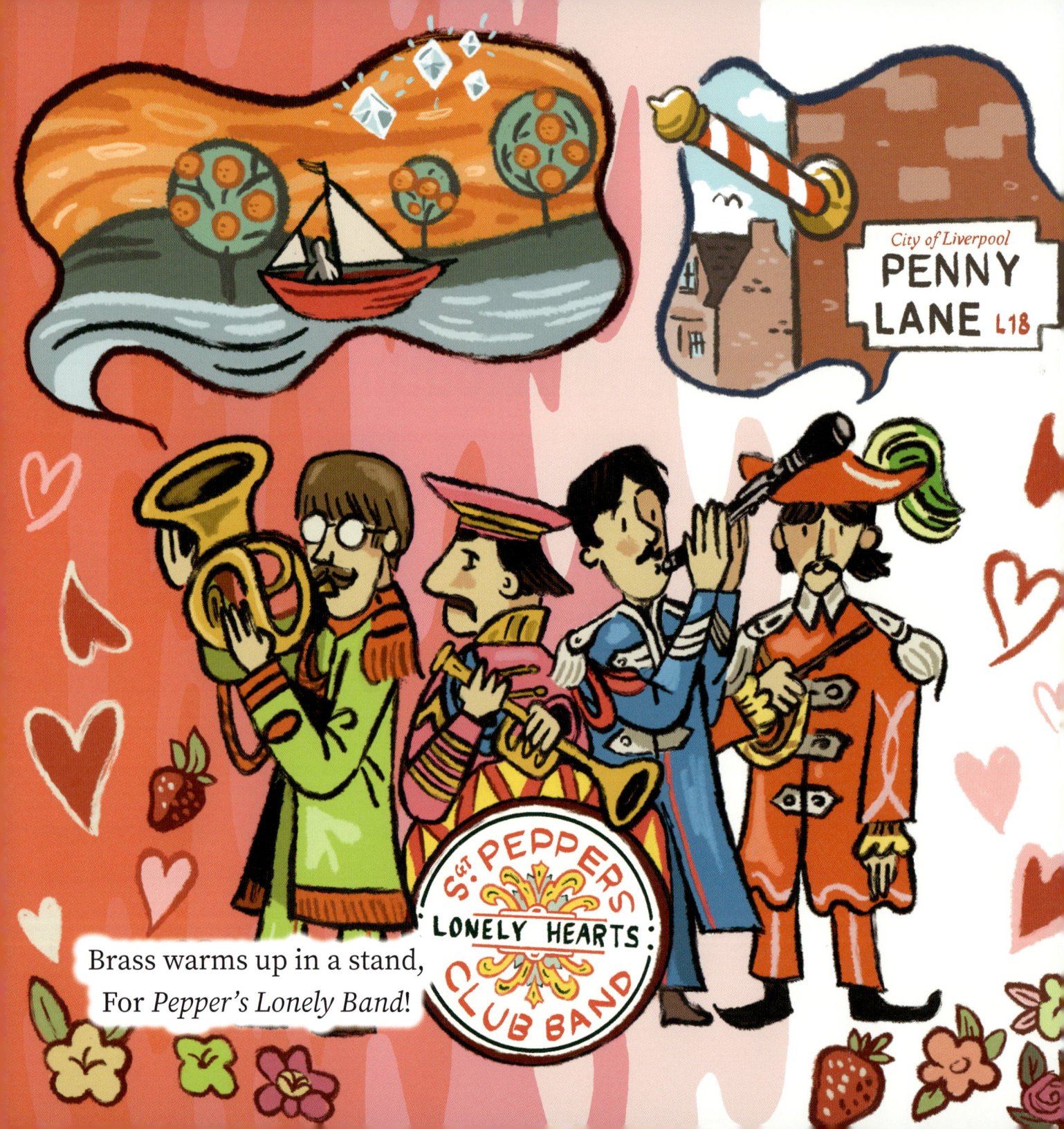

City of Liverpool
PENNY
LANE L18

S.GT PEPPERS
LONELY HEARTS
CLUB BAND

Brass warms up in a stand,
For *Pepper's Lonely Band!*

Sgt. Pepper's Lonely Hearts Club Band

So touring is behind them, you'd think that would be sad,
But better still to come, that is, I think it's not too bad.
The studio becomes the place where talents do sustain,
A taste of *Strawberry Fields* comes out, *Forever Penny Lane*.
A needle down, the sound it comes, brass warming in a stand,
A guitar chord, a beating drum, it's *Pepper's Lonely Band*.
She's Leaving Home, it's *Lucy's Sky*, they're sharper than a knife,
The astonishing crescendo; a fine *Day In The Life*.

These memories last forever,
A fine old *Mystery Tour*,
Getting Better, all the time,
Remember our Fab Four.

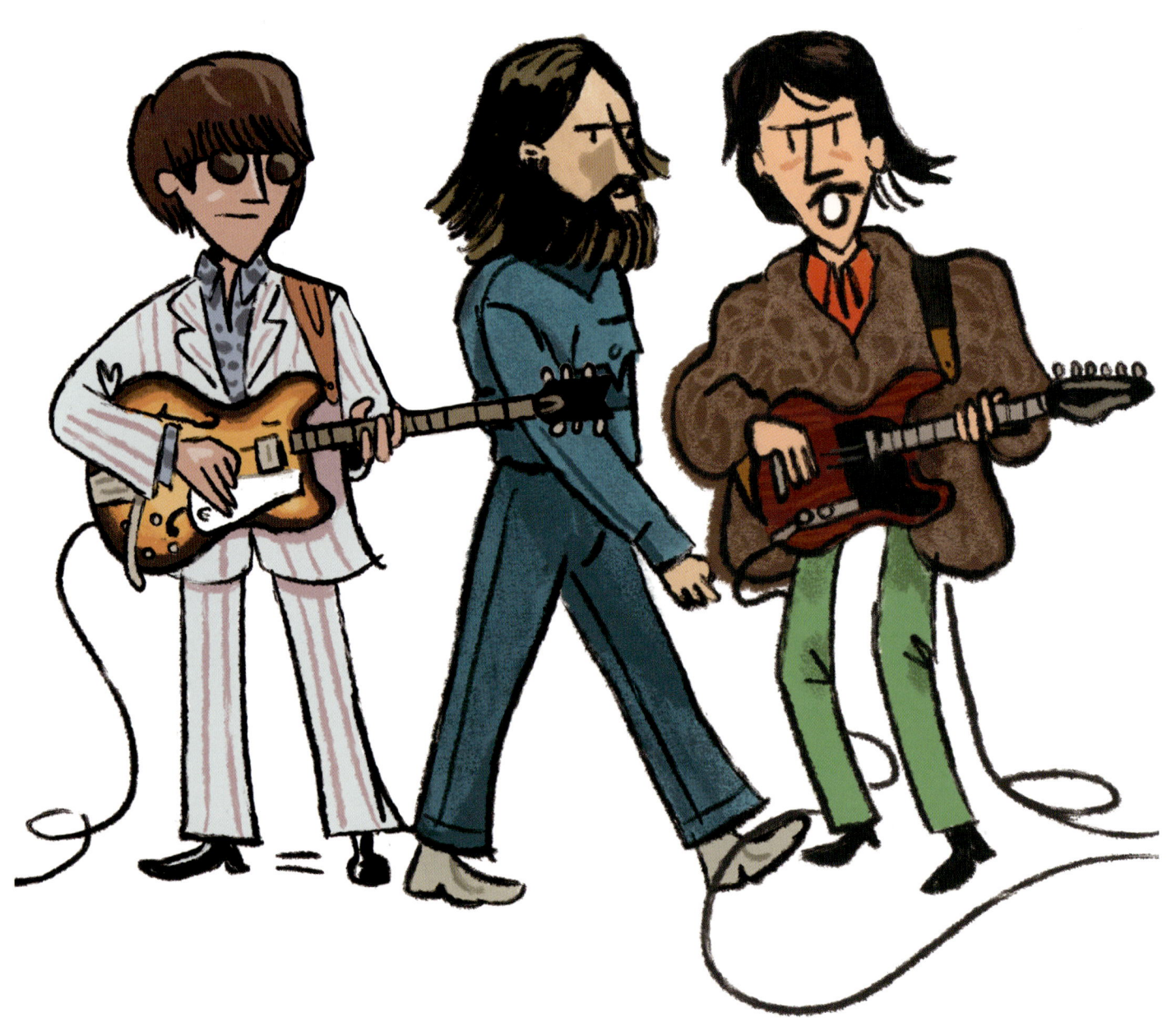

George Harrison was class!
And *All* these *Things Must Pass.*

George

The youngest one of all the group, the one with less to say,
But his guitar did gently talk, it *Wept* when he did play.
Handsome too, impressive; far better than good,
Even learns to play sitar, starts on *Norwegian Wood*.
Something says the songs he wrote are beyond criticism,
Along with a keen interest in Indian mysticism.
Funds *The Life Of Brian*, George Harrison was class,
Leaves us young, *My Sweet Lord*! *All* these *Things Must Pass*.

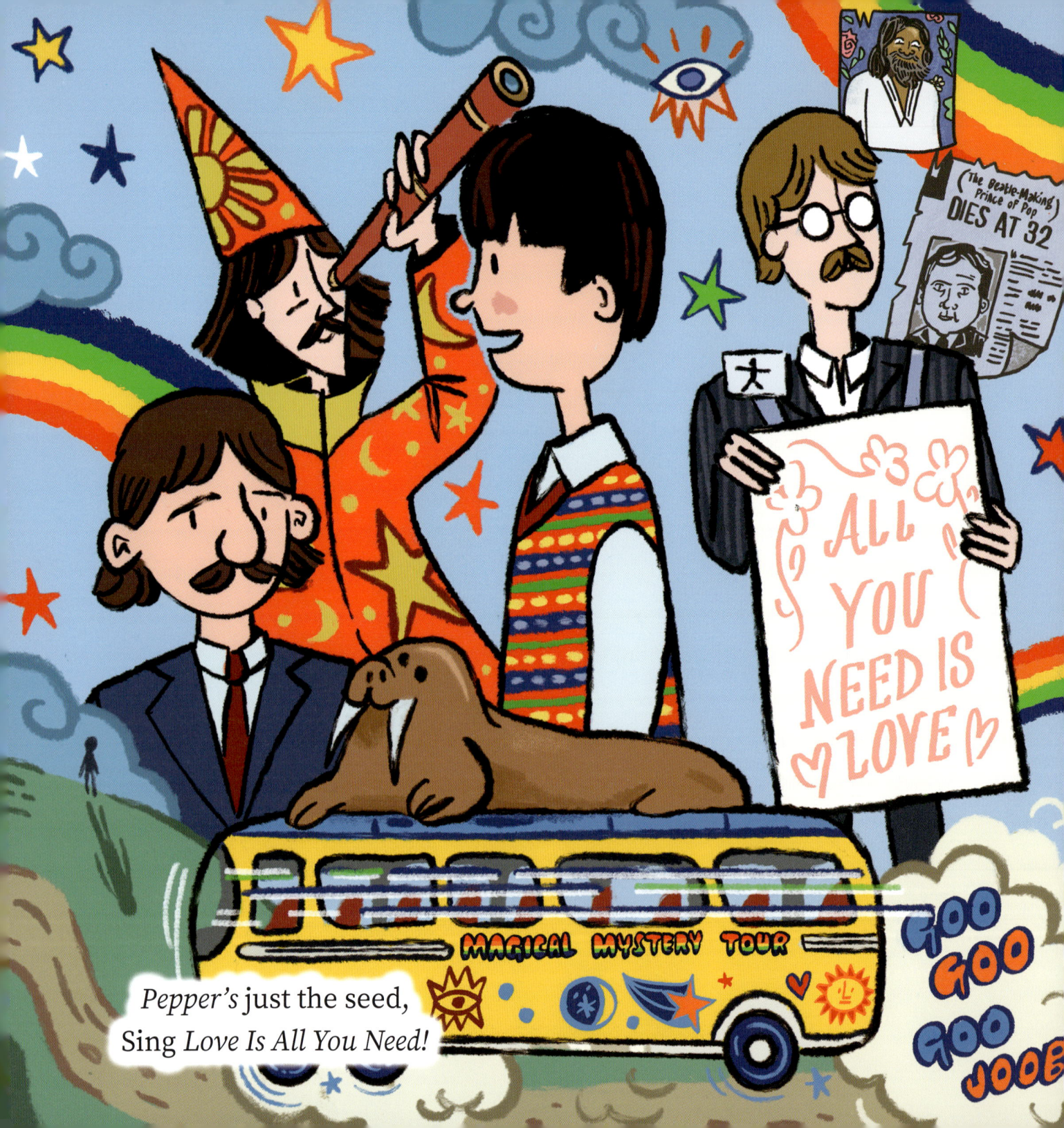

Pepper's just the seed,
Sing *Love Is All You Need!*

1967

The year it isn't over yet, *Pepper's* just the seed,
A TV-first across the globe sing *Love Is All You Need*.
A trip to Bangor, all Fab Four, each of them does wish he,
Could reach a higher plain of truth, helped by The Maharishi!
Brian Epstein's home alone, his life is far too brief,
The Beatles now must forge ahead, united in their grief.
With *Fools On Hills* and *Walruses*, a bus that does not stop,
They embark upon that *Magic Tour*; Paul wears a loud tank top!

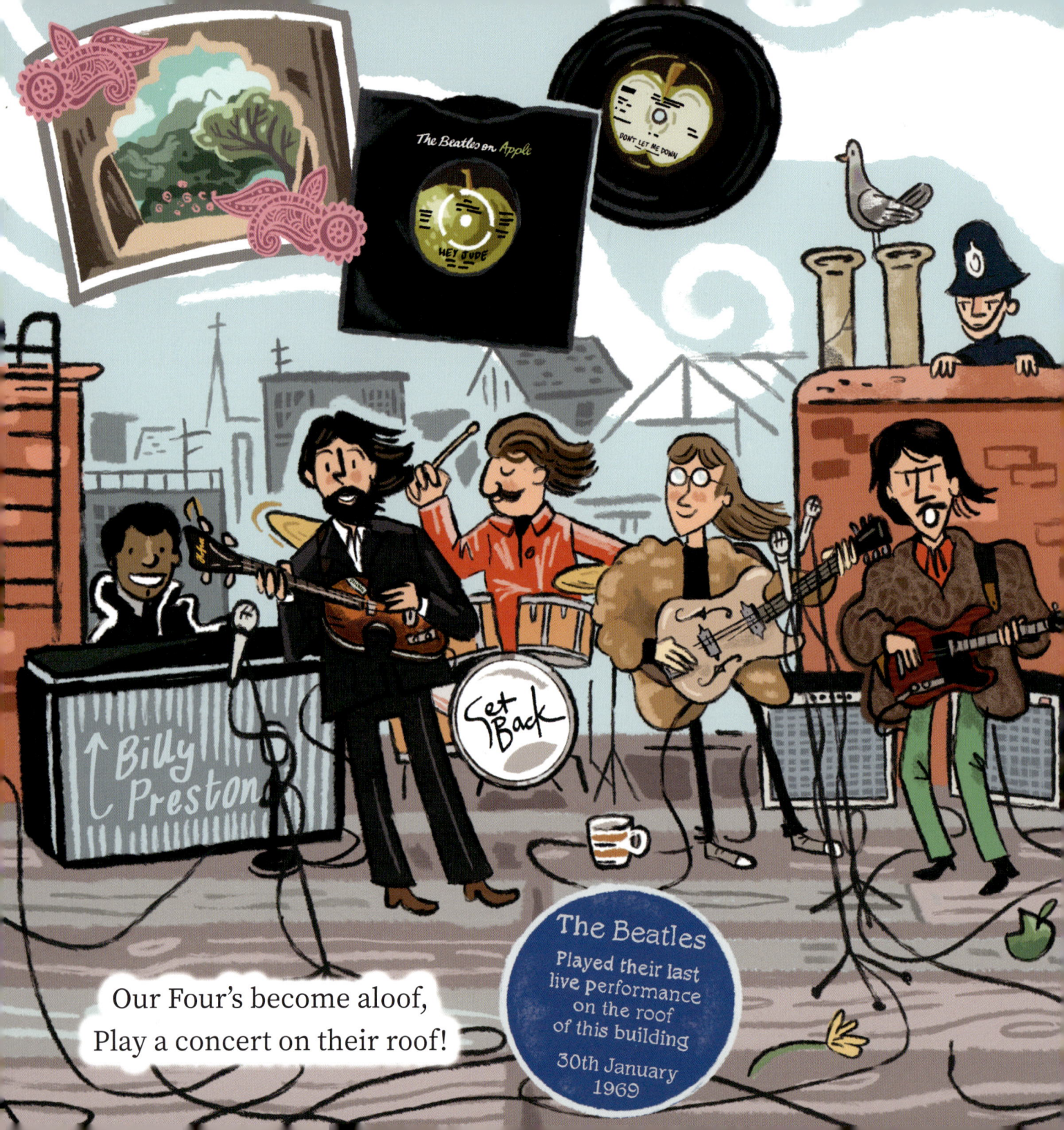

Our Four's become aloof,
Play a concert on their roof!

1968 to 1969

Hello, Goodbye to India, to meditate and write,
New songs for an album, its gatefold only white.
Songs of *Revolution*, each one a different mood,
One tune's now played every hour, you can't escape *Hey Jude*!
But the Apple Corps' quite sour now, the squabbling's sometimes silly,
The cameras roll to film them play with a keyboardist named Billy.
Dig It, they *Don't Let Me Down*, although they're quite aloof,
A brief *Get Back* to playing live: a concert on their roof!

These memories last forever,
A fine old *Mystery Tour*,
Good Night, Good Morning, Slumbers Gold,
Remember our Fab Four.

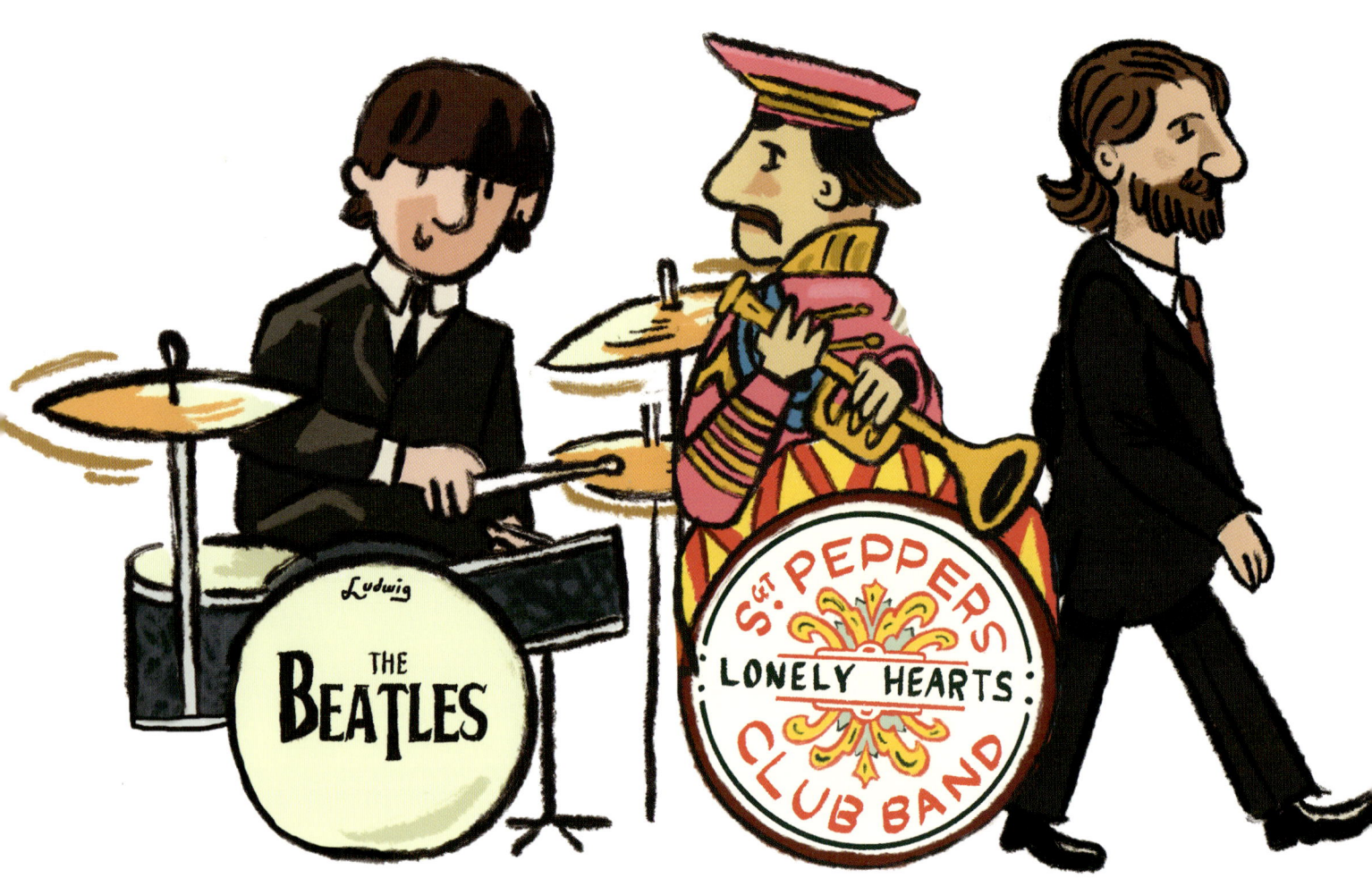

Our Ringo passed the test,
Replacing young Pete Best!

Ringo

We see him at the drumkit, his hair is flowing wild,
But Richard Starkey has a past, so sickly as a child.
Through Rory Storm and Hurricanes, our Ringo passed the test,
Asked to join in '62, replacing young Pete Best.
The solid man right at the back, he brought us all the joys,
Singing too, *A Little Help*, a *Submarine* and *Boys*.
Don't ignore his influence, to Mr Starr give thanks,
Later on the *Photograph* and all those Thomas the Tanks!

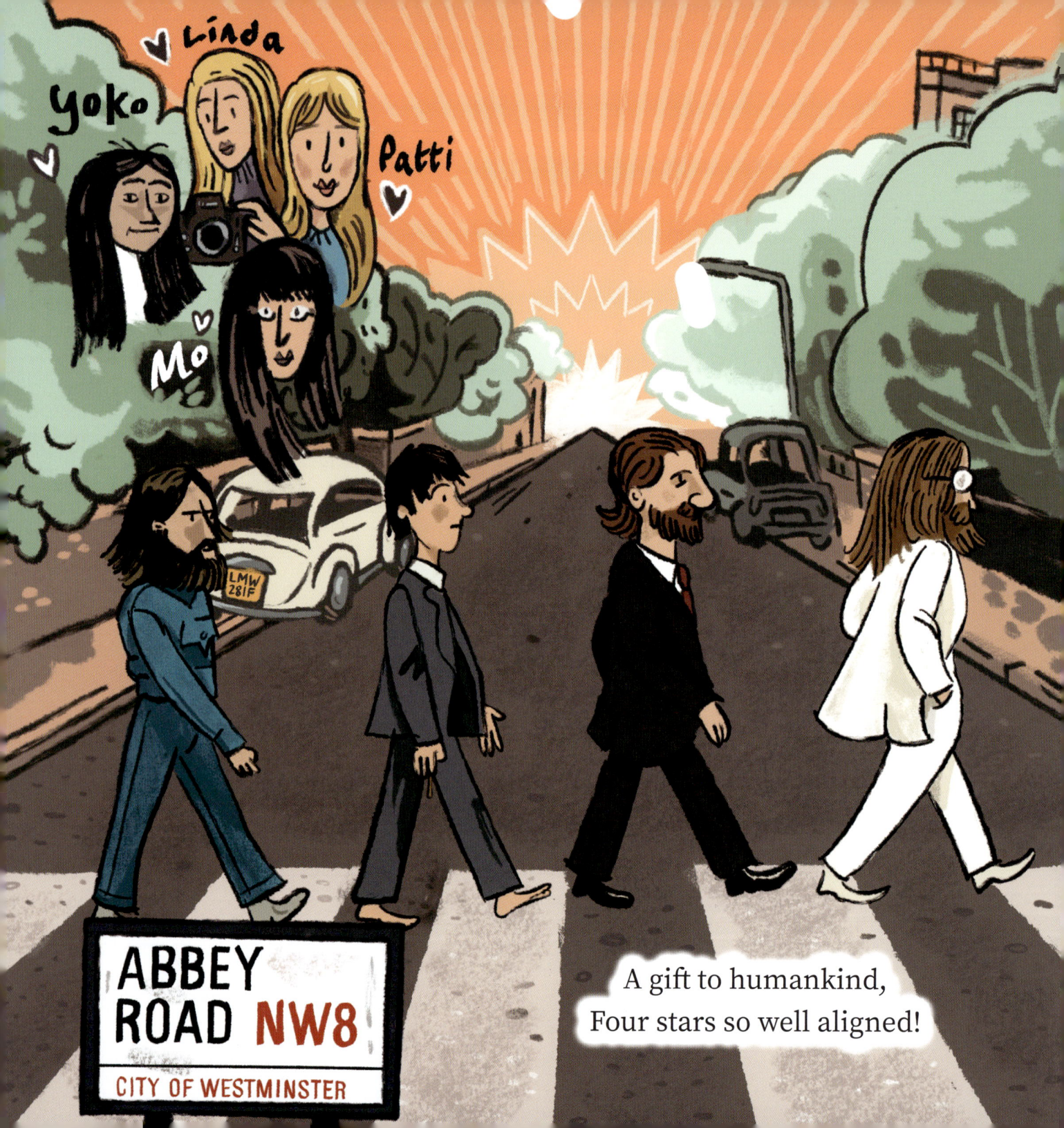

The End

Our heroes *Come Together*, for one last final run,
In *Abbey Road* their curtain call, watch! *Here Comes The Sun.*
Lawyers now, resentments brew, the bond is not so strong,
New wives, new lives, the mood is rife, *Weight Carried* far too long.
But history's not changeable, we know that wc were blessed,
We were there to witness the undisputed best.
We lived through Beatlemania, a gift to humankind,
And we look back to know we see four stars so well aligned.

These memories last forever,
A fine old *Mystery Tour*,
Let it Be and in *The End,*
Remember our Fab Four.

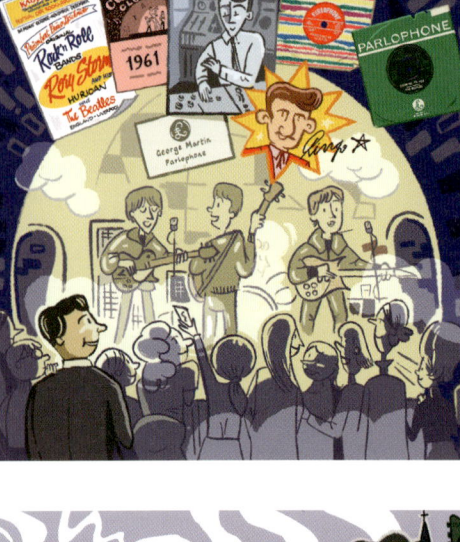
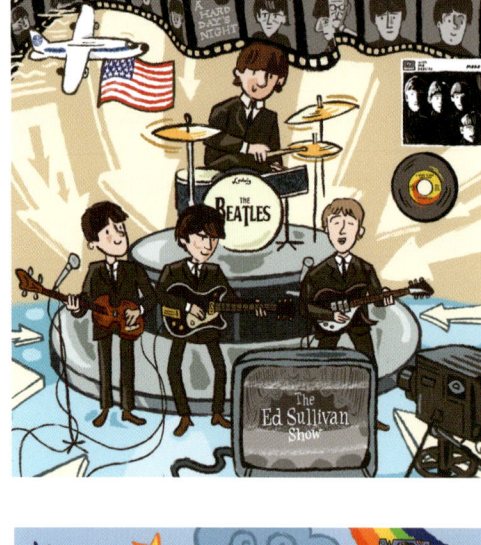
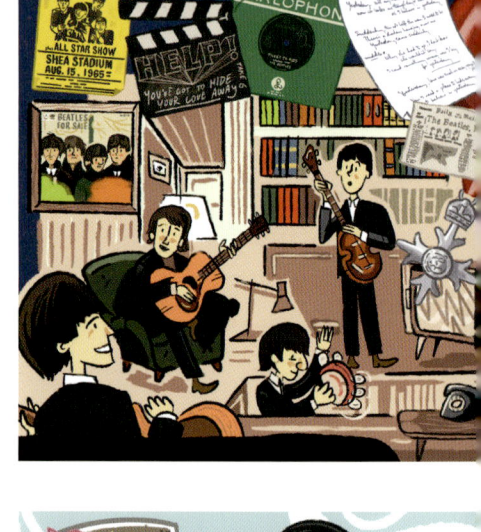
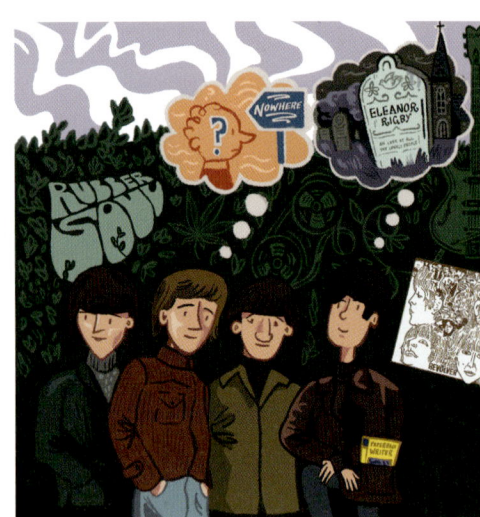
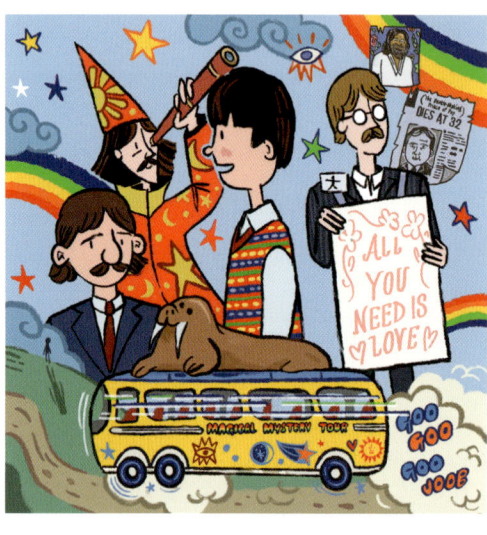
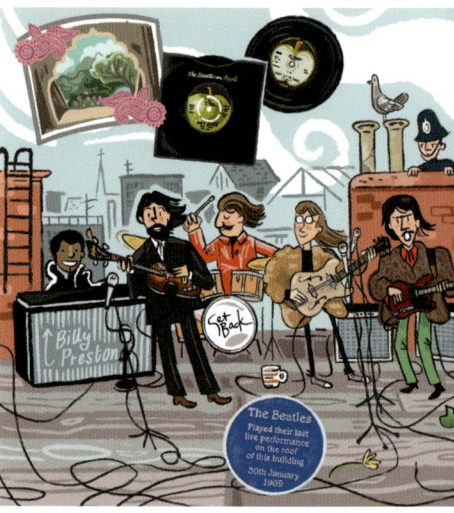
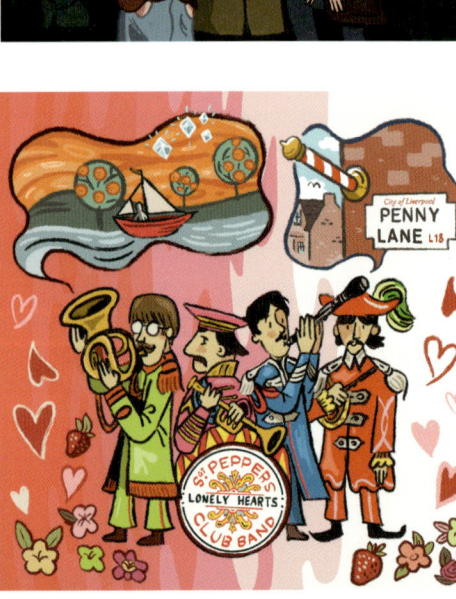
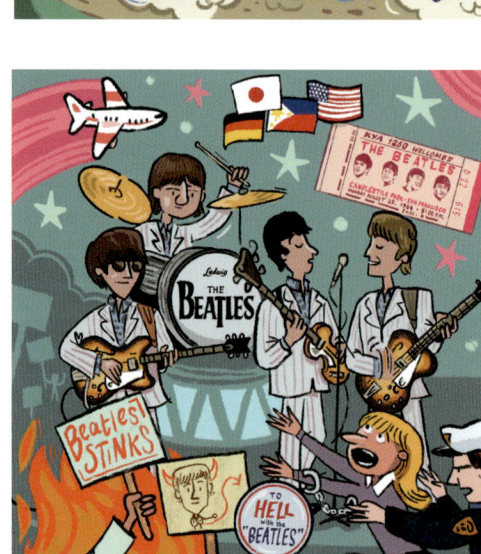
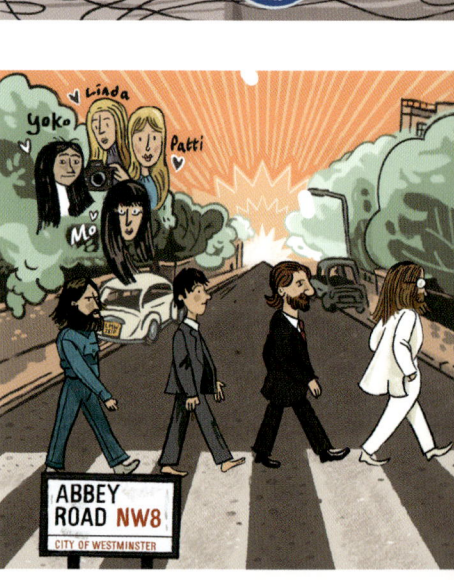

Exercises

To help cognition and to stimulate conversation

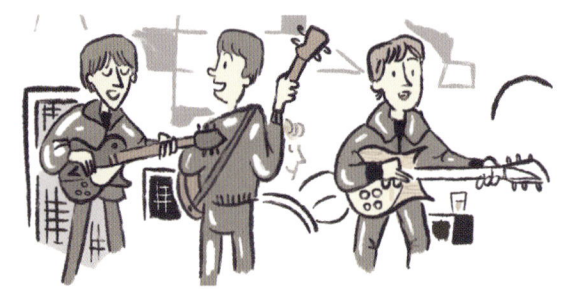

Just for fun – it's quiz time!

These questions are from the story and all the answers can be found in the book!
You get one mark for each with a total of thirteen to get. The answers are on page 58.

1960 to 1963 (page 9):

In which West German city did The Beatles play clubs like The Top Ten and the Kaiserkeller before they became famous?

    a.   Frankfurt

    b.   Hanover

    c.   Hamburg

1963 to 1964 (page 11):

What was the name of The Beatles' first movie?

    a.   *Help!*

    b.   *Yellow Submarine*

    c.   *A Hard Day's Night*

John (page 13):

Which guitar parts did John mainly play in The Beatles?

    a.   Rhythm

    b.   Bass

    c.   Lead

1964 to 1965 (page 15):

What honour did the Queen give The Beatles, which upset the establishment?

    a.   Knighthoods

    b.   MBEs

    c.   Freedom of Buckingham Palace

1965 to 1966 (page 17):

On which LP are the songs *Eleanor Rigby* and *Here, There And Everywhere*?

    a.   *Abbey Road*

    b.   *With The Beatles*

    c.   *Revolver*

Paul (page 19):

Paul is right-handed?

    a.   True

    b.   False

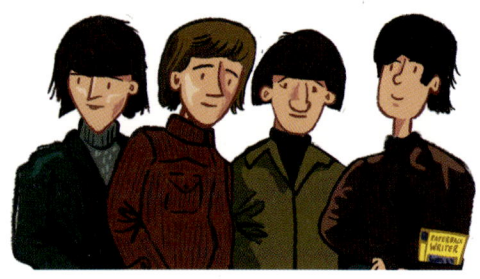

The end of touring (page 21):

Where was The Beatles' last concert of their final tour in 1966?

a.   Tokyo, Japan

b.   Candlestick Park, San Francisco, USA

c.   London, UK

Sgt. Pepper's Lonely Hearts Club Band (page 23):

What was the double A-sided single released shortly before *Sgt. Pepper's Lonely Hearts Club Band*?

a.   *Strawberry Fields Forever / Penny Lane*

b.   *Penny Lane / Being For The Benefit of Mr Kite!*

c.   *Lovely Rita / Strawberry Fields Forever*

George (page 25):

On which song recording did George first play sitar?

a.   *Something*

b.   *Norwegian Wood*

c.   *While My Guitar Gently Weeps*

1967 (page 27):

The Beatles performed which song on the first global satellite TV link-up show, called *Our World*?

a. *I Want To Hold Your Hand*

b. *All You Need Is Love*

c. *Let It Be*

1968 to 1969 (page 29):

Where did The Beatles perform a concert instead of a big stage show?

a. Ringo's garden

b. John's psychedelic Rolls Royce

c. Their roof (the Apple Corps' rooftop in Savile Row)

Ringo (page 31):

Who did Ringo replace as the drummer of The Beatles?

a. Charlie Watts

b. Pete Best

c. Keith Moon

The End (page 33):

Name the song on *Abbey Road: Here Comes The ...*

a. *Sun*

b. *Moon*

c. *Rain*

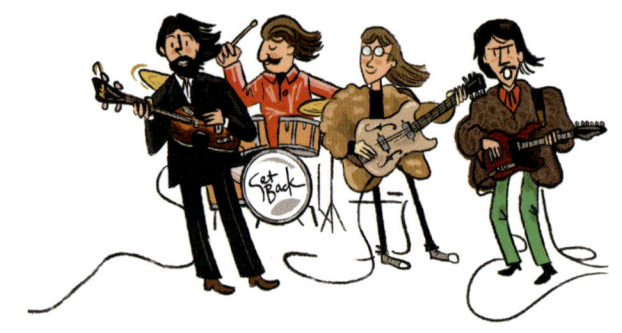

Some more ...

Here are some questions where the answers aren't in the book! Each question is worth one point (except the last, which is worth nine). There is a total of twenty points to get. The answers are on page 59.

1. **Which song starts with the line 'Well, she was just seventeen, you know what I mean'?**

   a.   *Roll Over Beethoven*

   b.   *Octopus's Garden*

   c.   *I Saw Her Standing There*

2. **Which Beatle released solo singles called *Woman* and *Imagine*?**

   a.   John

   b.   Paul

   c.   Ringo

3. **Who was The Beatles' bass player – who tragically died aged twenty-one in Hamburg – before Paul McCartney took over the role?**

a. Stuart Sutcliffe

b. John Entwistle

c. Bill Wyman

4. **At *The Royal Variety Performance* in 1963, John Lennon cheekily suggested that, 'the people in the cheaper seats clap your hands, and the rest of you, if you'd just rattle your ...' what?**

a. Champagne glasses!

b. Jewellery!

c. Servants!

5. **In 1982, Paul McCartney released a duet called *Ebony And Ivory* with which famous Motown singer?**

a. Smokey Robinson

b. Diana Ross

c. Stevie Wonder

6. **Which song includes the lines 'tangerine trees and marmalade skies', 'newspaper taxis appear on the shore' and 'the girl with kaleidoscope eyes'?**

   a. *Lucy In The Sky With Diamonds*

   b. *Get Back*

   c. *Paperback Writer*

7. **George Harrison recorded a hit single in 1987 called *Got My Mind Set On* ... what?**

   a. *The Taxman*

   b. *You*

   c. *Tom Petty*

8. **Which Beatles LP famously features a picture of The Fab Four crossing a road on the cover?**

   a. *With The Beatles*

   b. *Abbey Road*

   c. *The Beatles* (also known as *The White Album*)

9. **Complete the lyric: 'Will you still need me, will you still feed me ...'?**

   a. I'm starving!

   b. Some fish and finger pies

   c. When I'm sixty-four

10. Ringo is left-handed but plays the drums right-handed?

    a.   True

    b.   False

11. Which of these is not a song by Lennon and McCartney?

    a.   *Please Please Me*

    b.   *Paperback Writer*

    c.   *Long Tall Sally*

12. Between them, up to the present day, John, Paul, George and Ringo had *nine* wives! How many can you name (one point for each)?

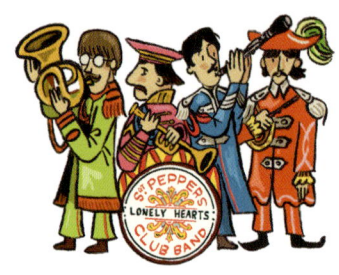

Did we know?

Some facts about The Beatles that aren't so well known!

? *Did we know* that on *The White Album* is a song called *Martha My Dear*, which Paul McCartney wrote about his Old English sheepdog, Martha!

? *Did we know* that John Lennon counted in the recording of *A Day In The Life*, on *Sgt. Pepper's Lonely Hearts Club Band*, with the words 'Sugar plum fairy; sugar plum fairy' instead of numbers!

? *Did we know* that the song *Dear Prudence* is written about actress Mia Farrow's sister, Prudence, who wouldn't come out of her dwellings when she was in India with The Beatles; hence 'Dear Prudence, won't you come out to play?'!

? *Did we know* that John Lennon's 'bigger than Jesus' quote came from a 1966 interview with journalist, Maureen Cleave, for the *London Evening Standard* newspaper. Nobody commented and there was no controversy in the UK. It was only when an American journalist picked up John's comments about more young people following The Beatles than were going to church that the outrage started!

Did we know that the song *Something* was written by George Harrison about his wife at the time, Pattie (née Boyd). *Wonderful Tonight* and *Layla* were also written about her – by Eric Clapton!

Did we know that the song titles *A Hard Day's Night* and *Tomorrow Never Knows* are 'Ringoisms' – strange phrases Ringo dropped into conversations that made no sense ... but somehow did make sense!

Did we know that when The Beatles appeared on *Morecambe and Wise*, Eric Morecambe referred to Ringo as 'Bongo'!

Did we know that when The Beatles appeared live on the Apple Corps' rooftop on 30 January 1969, it was their first live appearance since Candlestick Park in San Francisco on 29 August 1966 – two and a half years earlier – and the last time they ever played live!

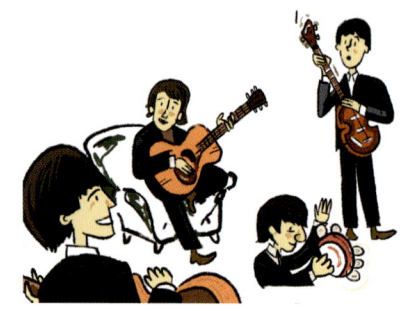

Let's chat

Here are some conversation topics for you to talk about – or even just think about. There's also some space to write notes if needed.

What other major events can you think of from the 1960s? Perhaps from sport, cinema, the news or even your own, or your family and friends', lives from that time?

What other music do you like? How many other artists can you name from the era when The Beatles were popular – groups, duets and solo acts?

Some of the big artists who influenced The Beatles were around in the rock 'n' roll 1950s – like Chuck Berry, Elvis Presley, Little Richard and Buddy Holly. Who do you like from that era and why?

Who is your favourite Beatle – John, Paul, George or Ringo?
What makes you say that?

What other major events can you think of from the 1960s? Perhaps from sport, cinema, the news or even your own, or your family and friends', lives from that time?

What other music do you like? How many other artists can you name from the era when The Beatles were popular – groups, duets and solo acts?

....

....

....

....

....

Some of the big artists who influenced The Beatles were around in the rock 'n' roll 1950s – like Chuck Berry, Elvis Presley, Little Richard and Buddy Holly. Who do you like from that era and why?

....

....

....

....

....

....

....

....

....

....

....

Who is your favourite Beatle – John, Paul, George or Ringo?
What makes you say that?

....

....

....

....

....

....

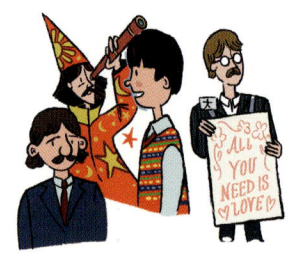

The Beatles' singles

Between October 1962 and March 1970, The Beatles released twenty-two singles (that's one every four months) … seventeen of them reached number one!

What are your top five?

1.

2.

3.

4.

5.

The full list

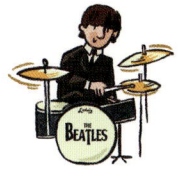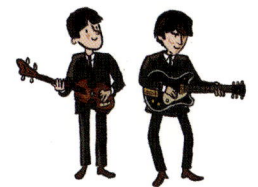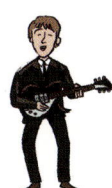

Single	UK release	Highest UK chart position
Love Me Do	October 1962	17
Please Please Me	January 1963	2
From Me To You	April 1963	1
She Loves You	August 1963	1
I Want To Hold Your Hand	November 1963	1
Can't Buy Me Love	March 1964	1
A Hard Day's Night	July 1964	1
I Feel Fine	November 1964	1
Ticket To Ride	April 1965	1
Help!	July 1965	1
(Double A-Side): *Day Tripper / We Can Work It Out*	December 1965	1
Paperback Writer	June 1966	1
(Double A-Side): *Eleanor Rigby / Yellow Submarine*	August 1966	1
(Double A-Side): *Strawberry Fields Forever / Penny Lane*	February 1967	2
All You Need Is Love	July 1967	1
Hello, Goodbye	November 1967	1
Lady Madonna	March 1968	1
Hey Jude	August 1968	1
Get Back	April 1969	1
The Ballad Of John And Yoko	May 1969	1
(Double A-Side): *Something / Come Together*	October 1969	4
Let It Be	March 1970	2
Free As A Bird	December 1995	2
Real Love	March 1996	4
Now And Then	November 2023	1

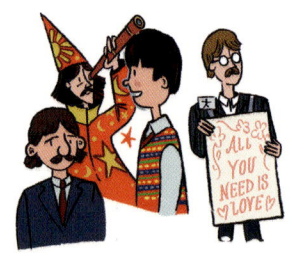

The Beatles' albums

Between March 1963 and May 1970, The Beatles released twelve studio albums in the UK. All but one reached number one in the UK album charts!

What are your top three?

1.
2.
3.

The full list

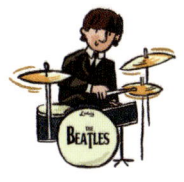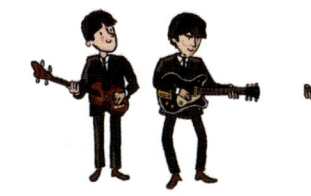

Album	Key songs from the album	UK release	Highest UK chart position
Please Please Me	*I Saw Her Standing There; Love Me Do; Twist And Shout*	March 1963	1
With The Beatles	*All My Loving; Roll Over Beethoven; I Wanna Be Your Man*	November 1963	1
A Hard Day's Night	*And I Love Her; Can't Buy Me Love; You Can't Do That*	July 1964	1
Beatles For Sale	*Rock And Roll Music; I'll Follow The Sun; Eight Days A Week*	December 1964	1
Help!	*You've Got To Hide Your Love Away; Ticket To Ride; Yesterday*	August 1965	1
Rubber Soul	*Drive My Car; Norwegian Wood; In My Life*	December 1965	1
Revolver	*Taxman; Eleanor Rigby; Tomorrow Never Knows*	August 1966	1
Sgt. Pepper's Lonely Hearts Club Band	*Lucy In The Sky With Diamonds; When I'm Sixty-Four; A Day In The Life*	May 1967	1
The Beatles ('The White Album')	*Back In The USSR; Ob-La-Di, Ob-La-Da; While My Guitar Gently Weeps*	November 1968	1
Yellow Submarine	*All Together Now; Hey Bulldog; All You Need Is Love*	January 1969	3
Abbey Road	*Come Together; Something; Here Comes The Sun*	September 1969	1
Let It Be	*Across The Universe; The Long And Winding Road; Get Back*	May 1970	1

All about me

In this section, you can share some things that are personal to you. It's great to do these things in twos if there's someone else who knows you well!

a picture of me

Name:
....

Date of birth:
....

Birthplace:
....

People who are important to me:
....

....

My favourite films:
....

....

My favourite music:
....

....

My favourite book:

....

....

My favourite food:

....

....

My favourite drink:

....

....

My favourite places:

....

....

Things that make me laugh:

....

....

Things that make me cry:

....

....

Scrapbook

A place to put pictures, newspaper or magazine clippings, tickets, drawings, notes
... or anything you like!

Just for fun – it's quiz time!
Answers

1960 to 1963:
c. Hamburg

1963 to 1964:
c. *A Hard Day's Night*

John:
a. Rhythm

1964 to 1965:
b. MBEs

1965 to 1966:
c. *Revolver*

Paul:
b. False

End of touring:
b. Candlestick Park

Sgt. Pepper's Lonely Hearts Club Band:
a. *Strawberry Fields Forever / Penny Lane*

George:
b. *Norwegian Wood*

1967:
b. *All You Need Is Love*

1968 to 1969:
c. Their roof

Ringo:
b. Pete Best

The End:
a. *Sun*

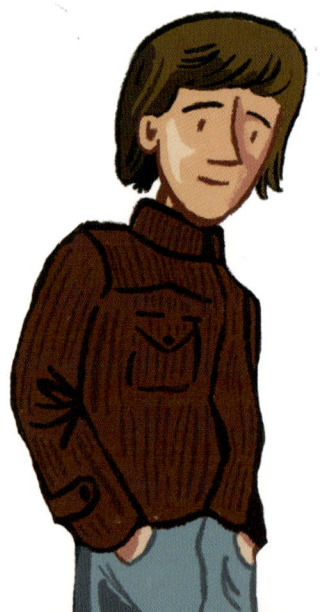

Some more ...
Answers

1.
c. *I Saw Her Standing There*

2.
a. John

3.
a. Stuart Sutcliffe

4.
b. Jewellery

5.
c. Stevie Wonder

6.
a. *Lucy In The Sky With Diamonds*

7.
b. You

8.
b. *Abbey Road*

9.
c. When I'm sixty-four

10.
a. True

11.
c. *Long Tall Sally*

12.
John – Cynthia (Powell) and Yoko (Ono); Paul – Linda (Eastman), Heather (Mills) and Nancy (Shevell); George – Pattie (Boyd) and Olivia (Arias); Ringo – Maureen (Cox) and Barbara (Bach)

Supporters' guide

This section is for the loved ones or carers of people living with dementia or other cognitive difficulties. If you're the carer or a loved one of the person reading this book, you can enjoy it too!

Here are some useful hints and tips to
make sure everyone gets the most out of their Cognitive Book.

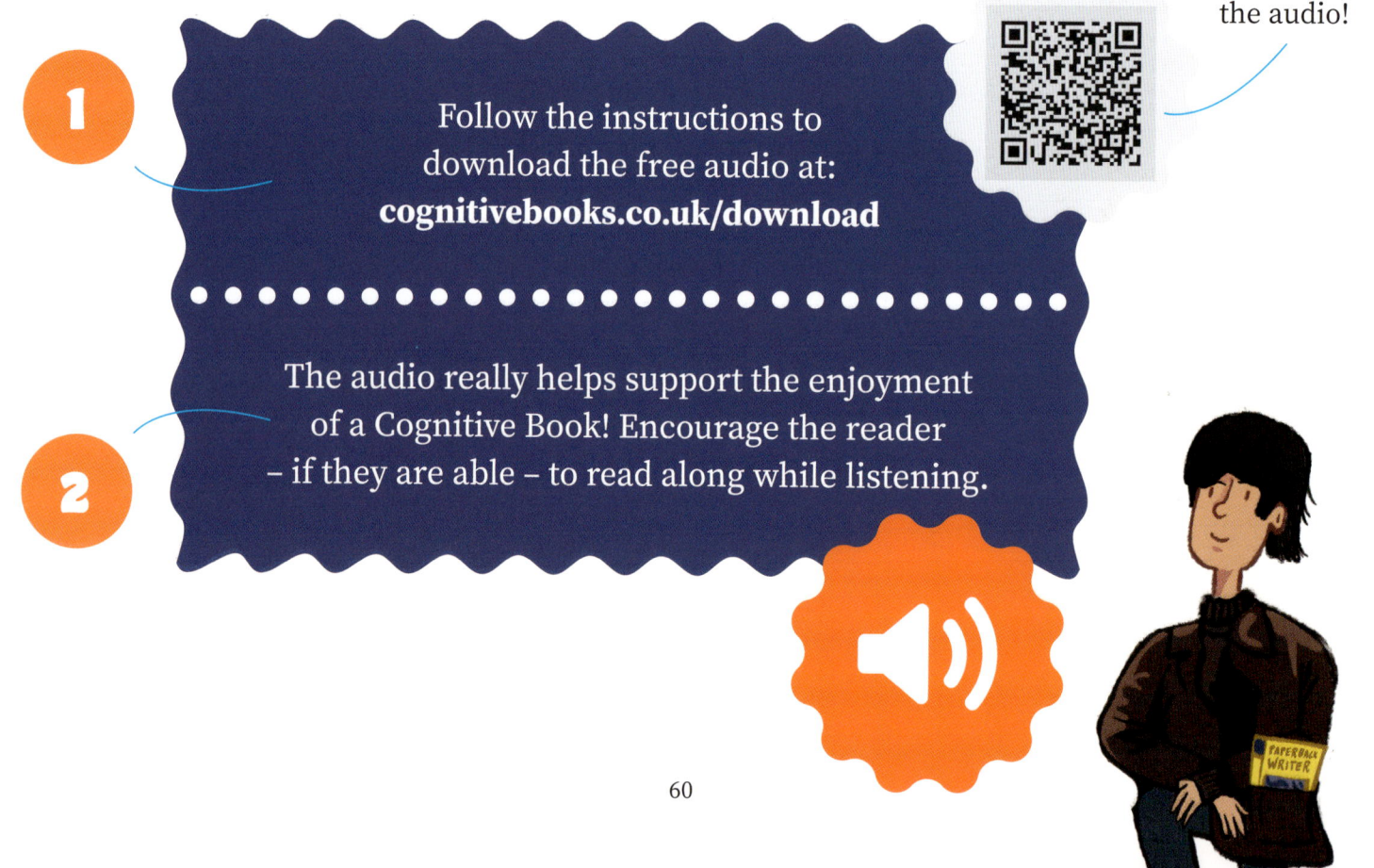

Scan here for the audio!

1

Follow the instructions to download the free audio at:
cognitivebooks.co.uk/download

2

The audio really helps support the enjoyment of a Cognitive Book! Encourage the reader – if they are able – to read along while listening.

3 Don't leave this book in amongst other books – like on a bookshelf or in a pile by the bedside.

Always leave the book somewhere it's frequently to hand and easy to access – the armrest of the sofa or a table near where the reader regularly sits, or the bedside table if they like to read at night, for example.

4

5 For those finding reading more difficult these days, it might be better to stick to the left-hand page of each spread to enjoy the simpler text and vibrant illustrations.

Many readers will be able to explore a Cognitive Book largely on their own – the full text on the right-hand page of each spread will often be accessible to them.

6

7 Pages 35 to 59 contain exercises you can work on together. Try to support the reader in answering the quiz questions (pages 36-43), give prompts for the 'Let's chat' questions (page 46), and help them complete the 'All about me' and 'Scrapbook' sections (pages 54-57).

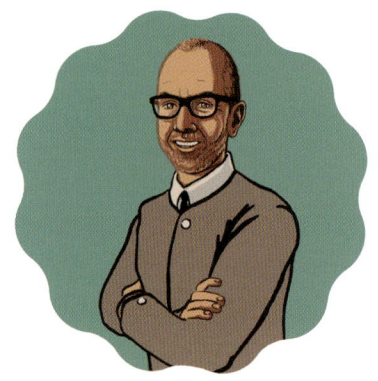

Cognitive Books are enjoyed by everyone.

They've also been tried and tested on people living with dementia. I didn't start writing Cognitive Books for people with dementia. I wrote for my Dad, Brian. It just so happens he *is* living with dementia. I wanted to create something he'd enjoy today but, equally, something he'd have taken pleasure in reading twenty years ago.

After testing the books with Alzheimer's Society, we realised how many people with and without dementia would enjoy them! We hope you do too.

Sign up to our mailing list at cognitivebooks.co.uk to discover future titles.

Happy reading!

Matt Singleton
Author and director of Cognitive Books
cognitivebooks.co.uk

Explore the wonderful world of The Beatles!

 **YouTube:** You can watch classic and new footage, and listen to their music at The Beatles' YouTube channel: Just scan the QR code or visit **bit.ly/cogbeatlesyoutube**

 **Spotify:** If you have a Spotify account, why not download the playlist of all songs mentioned in this book? Just scan the QR code or visit **spoti.fi/3MN20tO**

 **Compact Disc / Vinyl:** If you don't have an account, we recommend The Beatles 1962-1966 ('The Red Album') and The Beatles 1967-1970 ('The Blue Album'). These have been remixed and expanded in 2023. Just scan the QR code or visit: **bit.ly/cogbeatlesredblue**

All links are correct at the time of going to print.

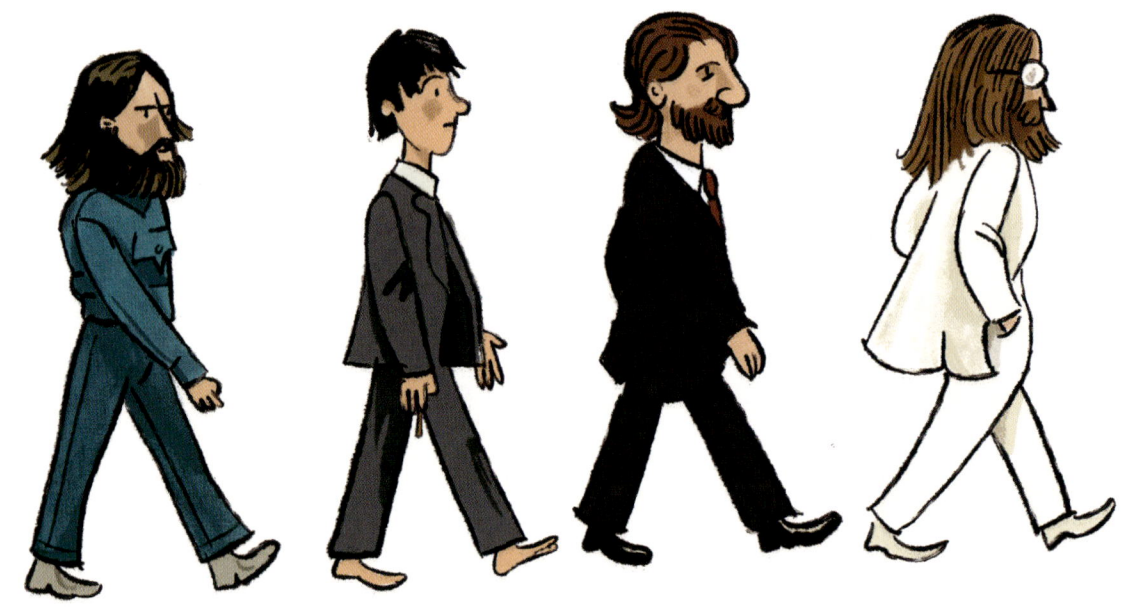

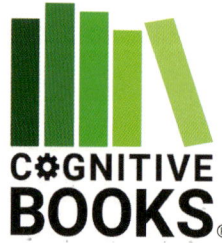